Everyone with a relative or friend suffering from Alzheimer's disease or dementia MUST read this book.

Millions of Alzheimer's Patients Have Been Misdiagnosed (And Could Be Cured)

D1460630

Dr Vernon Coleman MB ChB DSc FRSA

The author: Vernon Coleman is a qualified doctor who worked as a
GP principal in England. He has organised many successful medical
campaigns. For example, after a 15 year campaign (which started in
1973), he eventually persuaded the British Government to introduce
stricter controls governing the prescribing of benzodiazepine
tranquillisers. ('Dr Vernon Coleman's articles, to which I refer with
approval, raised concern about these important matters,' said the
Parliamentary Secretary for Health in the House of Commons in
1988.) Dr Coleman has given evidence to committees at the House
of Commons and House of Lords. He is a former editor of the *British
Clinical Journal*, has contributed articles and columns to leading
publications around the world and has lectured doctors and nurses on
a variety of medical matters. He is the best-selling author of over
100 books which have sold more than two million copies in the UK
and have been translated into 25 languages. For more information
please see www.vernoncoleman.com

In memory of Kathleen Alberta Coleman

Dedicated to Donna Antoinette Coleman, who cares.
With all my love and with my thanks.

Summary

Other than Alzheimer's disease, idiopathic normal pressure hydrocephalus is the commonest cause of dementia. It affects millions. The diagnosis is missed more than 80% of the time. Millions of patients with Alzheimer's disease or dementia have been wrongly diagnosed. They have idiopathic normal pressure hydrocephalus and they can be treated and cured.

Contents

Introduction

The failure to diagnose normal pressure hydrocephalus is one of the biggest health scandals of the last 50 years.

Millions of patients have been wrongly diagnosed as suffering from Alzheimer's Disease, other forms of dementia or Parkinson's disease and, since there is no known cure for any of these disorders, they have been more or less abandoned by the medical profession and by society.

Studies suggest that between five and ten per cent of all individuals diagnosed as suffering from Alzheimer's Disease or dementia have been misdiagnosed and are suffering from normal pressure hydrocephalus; a disorder which can produce similar symptoms – but which can be treated.

Around the world there are estimated to be nearly 50 million people suffering from dementia or Alzheimer's disease. One half of all the patients admitted to nursing homes are suffering from dementia of one sort or another. Millions of other patients who have been diagnosed with dementia of one kind or another are being looked after by their families. Many family members have had to abandon their jobs and their normal lives in order to find the necessary time. Millions more patients have been dumped in hospitals and nursing homes where they sit or lie, waiting to die. No one knows how many millions of undiagnosed individuals are struggling to cope with dementia, either alone or with the help of relatives, friends and neighbours.

Despite many promises there is still no cure for dementia or Alzheimer's disease, nor is there any sign of one, but there is clear evidence that many so-called dementia sufferers are actually suffering from something quite different – a health problem which can be cured.

Most cases of dementia cannot be treated (though there are a number of things which can be done to slow down the pace at which the disease develops) but there is one particular cause of dementia which can be treated: idiopathic normal pressure hydrocephalus.

If a friend or relative is diagnosed with dementia then you should not accept the diagnosis until doctors have confirmed that the patient is not suffering from idiopathic normal pressure hydrocephalus – a disorder which is commonly misdiagnosed as Alzheimer's disease, dementia or Parkinson's disease. It is important to rule out idiopathic normal pressure hydrocephalus because this disorder can be treated. And if the treatment is started early then the outlook is good.

Idiopathic normal pressure hydrocephalus is bizarrely under-researched, under-diagnosed and under-treated. There is almost certainly no disease affecting large numbers of people which is less understood.

Doctors certainly do not take the disorder as seriously as they should. Within the medical profession it is known (when it is known at all) as the 'wet, wacky and wobbly disease' – more a childhood term of abuse than a phrase redolent with respect.

Organisations which specialise in caring for the elderly are often appallingly ignorant about the disease, as are health websites.

On the internet, I asked the questions 'Why are old people unstable?' and 'Why do old people fall so often?' and none of the first several dozen responses mentioned 'idiopathic normal pressure hydrocephalus'. In the UK, the NHS Choices website devotes less than 70 words to the disease and describes the condition as 'uncommon' which is manifest nonsense since it affects millions and is undoubtedly the commonest treatable cause of major disability and mental incapacity among the elderly.

Researchers are not interested in investigating the disease because a cure is already available and, since there is no need for a 'wonder drug' there are not going to be any big, fat grants from drug companies. And doctors are not interested in diagnosing or treating the disease because it invariably involves older patients, and doctors are encouraged by governments (and much of society) not to take much interest in elderly patients.

If you made a list of the 100 commonest, potentially fatal but most easily cured medical conditions which are most often mistakenly diagnosed as something else, then idiopathic normal pressure hydrocephalus would be top of the list.

There is no doubt that a large percentage of the patients who are said to have died of Alzheimer's disease were suffering from normal pressure hydrocephalus. Alzheimer's disease causes dementia and a loss of mental abilities but (despite the fact that it is officially regarded as a major killer – in the US it is said to be the fifth commonest killer of people over the age of 65) there is no real reason why Alzheimer's disease should result in death. When patients are said to have died of Alzheimer's disease, or some other form of dementia, they will have usually died of pneumonia or some other infection which has been deliberately left untreated. A patient who has genuinely died as a direct result of their dementia, without an infection or any other complication, will have probably died of idiopathic normal pressure hydrocephalus which was not diagnosed but which caused death by compressing, damaging and destroying many different parts of the brain.

The only things we know for certain are that idiopathic normal pressure hydrocephalus is terribly common, it produces devastating results, it is usually mistaken for something else and it is treatable. Patients who have been stuck in bed or in wheelchairs can, after treatment, get up and walk. They can resume their lives; talking and enjoying work and hobbies. Patients who have been abandoned have their lives back again.

A diagnosis of dementia (whether Alzheimer's or any other variety of dementia) can be devastating to a patient and to family and friends. But that diagnosis is often wrong. And if the correct diagnosis is idiopathic normal pressure hydrocephalus then the true cause of the dementia is treatable.

Chapter One

What is idiopathic normal pressure hydrocephalus?

Under normal circumstances, the space between the brain and the skull is filled with cerebrospinal fluid; a substance which is produced within the spaces of the brain, circulates in and around the brain and is gradually reabsorbed. In normal circumstances, the fluid is produced in the same quantities as it is being reabsorbed. The cerebrospinal fluid, which also surrounds the spinal cord, is there primarily to protect the brain in case of injury.

In the condition known as normal pressure hydrocephalus, the fluid is not reabsorbed as fast as it is produced.

When there is too much cerebrospinal fluid in and around the brain, the liquid accumulates in the ventricles – the spaces within the brain – and the brain is put under pressure, being pushed outwards. The result of this unusual pressure is that the brain is compressed and damaged in a variety of ways. The symptoms and signs of damage will depend upon the area of the brain affected. If the problem is not treated then the damage to the brain will be irreversible.

Logically, one might expect that with too much fluid in a confined space there would be an increase in fluid pressure. By definition, this does not happen with normal pressure hydrocephalus. The intracranial pressure is normal and the increased amount of fluid dilates the ventricular system. If a scan is done, the ventricles usually look dilated. However, even when patients have magnetic resonance imaging (MRI) of the brain, or computerised tomography (CT), the wrong diagnosis can still be made because doctors who are not aware of normal pressure hydrocephalus will probably assume not that the ventricles have become larger but that the brain has become smaller as a result of cerebral atrophy.

There are two types of normal pressure hydrocephalus – secondary and idiopathic. Secondary normal pressure hydrocephalus can be caused by a variety of external problems including a head injury, a tumour, an infection or a bleed. But it is idiopathic normal pressure hydrocephalus which I am most concerned with here. This type of normal pressure hydrocephalus occurs with no underlying cause – it just happens.

Idiopathic normal pressure hydrocephalus, which was first described in 1965 by Salomon Hakim Dow and Raymond Delacy Adams, does not appear to be any commoner in men than in women or in women than in men and there is not as yet any evidence showing whether it is especially likely to affect any particular racial or ethnic groups. Although it can affect people of any age, it does, however, seem to be most commonly seen among patients in their 60s or older and it is this which results in patients being so often misdiagnosed as suffering from Alzheimer's disease.

'There are no cures for many types of dementia. But there are some treatable forms of dementia and normal pressure hydrocephalus is one of them,' said Ann Marie Flannery, a neurosurgeon at Women's and Children's Hospital in Lafayette, Louisiana, USA.

Chapter Two

What are the symptoms of idiopathic normal pressure hydrocephalus?

The initial, main symptom is often a curious, wide legged, unsteady walk. The patient's feet seem to stick to the floor, and have to be dragged up in order to make the next step. Patients adopt a wide legged gait in an attempt to make themselves more stable but they are, nevertheless, often unstable and may fall. Indeed, falling is a common problem with patients suffering from idiopathic normal pressure hydrocephalus and in any elderly person who falls frequently, the possible diagnosis of idiopathic normal pressure hydrocephalus should be placed quite high up on the list of possible causes.

Sadly, it is still the case that many leading health websites do not even mention normal pressure hydrocephalus as a possible cause of falls though the disorder should be listed towards the top of any such list, together with balance problems and drug side effects.

Since time is of the essence in diagnosing idiopathic normal pressure hydrocephalus, this disorder should always be considered very early on when a patient with dementia also falls.

Simply dismissing falls as 'an inevitable part of ageing', as some doctors are prone to do, is grossly irresponsible and unprofessional. Falling is not associated with any of the other common dementias, such as Alzheimer's disease.

The gait disturbance tends to get steadily worse as the amount of fluid increases and the ventricles within the brain expand. When the ventricles expand, they put pressure on the part of the nervous system which descends into the spinal cord.

In the early stages of idiopathic normal pressure hydrocephalus, the gait disturbance will probably be mild and result in the patient being unsteady and having impaired balance, particularly when trying to walk up and down stairs or steps or even kerbs. The patient will probably also complain that their legs feel weak, though there will probably be no explanation for this.

As the disease progresses, so the gait steadily gets worse. The patient will not lift their feet properly when walking and will walk very slowly. It is because of the gait disturbance that normal pressure hydrocephalus is often misdiagnosed as Parkinson's disease.

The tendency to fall is so common in idiopathic normal pressure hydrocephalus that it is, I think, reasonable to say that if a patient falls a good deal and suffers from some form of dementia then a diagnosis of idiopathic normal pressure hydrocephalus must be considered.

In the final stages of the disease, patients may be unable to walk, then unable to stand and finally even unable to turn over when lying in bed.

The second symptom is dementia, a chronic disorder of the mental processes which is caused by some brain disease or injury and which is characterised by mental disorders, personality changes and impaired reasoning. And, once again, this is why idiopathic normal pressure hydrocephalus is so often misdiagnosed as Alzheimer's disease, or some other cause of dementia.

The dementia in idiopathic normal pressure hydrocephalus usually involves the frontal lobe (because of the situation of the swelling ventricles within the brain) and patients will usually appear slow-witted, forgetful and apathetic. There may be an absence of mood (patients are neither happy when they might be expected to be happy nor sad when sadness might be appropriate) and patients often have difficulty in speaking.

The first sign of the dementia associated with this disease is often difficulty in planning, organising or putting things in order. The patient may also have difficulty in paying attention and in thinking in an abstract way.

Patients may lose interest in daily activities, they forget names and things to be done, they have difficulty in dealing with routine tasks and their short-term memory may be poor. (One sufferer complained that he could no longer read a book because when he tried he could not remember what had happened 10 pages earlier.)

Although this symptom is usually placed second chronologically, it may be noticeable much earlier in some patients. I suspect that the reason the mental problems are not recognised or recorded may often be because relatives and friends don't know what to look for, don't register subtle changes as being indicative of any underlying pathology and may dismiss changes as being simply consequences of 'old age'.

It is important to remember that dementia is not a disease but a consequence of some underlying disease. And it is vital to remember that although the dementia associated with idiopathic normal pressure hydrocephalus may appear similar, in superficial terms, to the dementia associated with Alzheimer's disease the two underlying disorders are quite different entities. There is, sadly, no cure for Alzheimer's disease at the moment but there is a remarkably effective and relatively simple cure available for idiopathic normal pressure hydrocephalus. To describe idiopathic normal pressure hydrocephalus as a variation of Alzheimer's disease (as I have seen done) is as nonsensical as describing heart disease as a type of cancer.

The final symptom to occur is often urinary incontinence.

Patients tend to have an increased sense of urgency (they suddenly need to urinate) but in the later stages, as the frontal lobe damage increases, they become indifferent to the consequences, and genuine urinary incontinence may result. In some cases, the urinary incontinence may occur quite early on in the disease. Some patients also develop faecal incontinence.

Mainstream medical textbooks do not include headache as a significant symptom in this condition but it can occur and it seems perfectly reasonable that it should. After all, the brain is being compressed and squashed against the skull and the eyes are under constant pressure. It would be rather unlikely if patients with this condition did not have, at the very least, an uncomfortable feeling in their heads.

Patients may have difficulty in focussing their eyes and occasionally, towards the end of the patient's life, the eyes may bulge as the pressure of fluid builds up.

Whatever symptoms may occur they tend to progress with time, sometimes slowly and sometimes quite quickly. Careful questioning of the patient may reveal that symptoms have been present for months or even years before a doctor was consulted. By then the patient may have, to a certain extent, become accustomed to their disability and the chances are high that they themselves will have learned to regard the difficulty in walking, the slowness of thought or the incontinence as an inevitable consequence of ageing. In many cases it is only when there is a critical loss of function, or a disability which dramatically affects the patient's independence, which leads to the patient seeking medical advice. At that point, the chances are high that the only solution on offer will be a bed in a nursing home or hospice or a suggestion that a relative should take over and provide accommodation and care.

The symptoms associated with normal pressure hydrocephalus do vary a good deal. The one constant factor seems to be the delay in making the diagnosis. Time and time again patients and relatives will report that it took years for an accurate diagnosis to be made and that even then it was only after the patient had seen a good many doctors. The evidence now suggests that in 80% of patients the correct diagnosis is never made.

Chapter Three

How common is idiopathic normal pressure hydrocephalus?

Idiopathic normal pressure hydrocephalus has been so little investigated that it is difficult to be certain how common it really is but there are three ways to tackle this vital question. All these methods make it very clear that idiopathic normal pressure hydrocephalus is far more common than most doctors believe. (A large proportion of doctors, including a surprising number of neurologists and psychiatrists are quite unfamiliar with the disorder.)

First, a study in Japan showed that idiopathic normal pressure hydrocephalus affects a far higher number of individuals than was historically considered possible or likely. Since there are no genetic or racial variations in the incidence of the disease, the figures can be applied globally.

The Japanese researchers investigated 567 individuals aged 65 and older and found seven patients with idiopathic normal pressure hydrocephalus. The researchers conclude 'the prevalence of possible idiopathic normal pressure hydrocephalus to be 1.4%' among individuals aged 65 and older.

When researchers in Sweden investigated the prevalence of probable idiopathic normal pressure hydrocephalus in a population of 65 years and older, they found the incidence to be 4%, with a higher proportion of men than women being diagnosed with the disease.

In the UK in 2016, there are approximately 10 million people aged 65 or older. If we use the Japanese figures for the UK's population then it would seem that there are currently around 140,000 people in the UK with normal pressure hydrocephalus. In the US, where there are considerably more than 40 million people aged 65 or older, the Japanese figures would suggest that there are around 560,000 people suffering from normal pressure hydrocephalus. If we use the Swedish figures then it suggests that there are currently 400,000 people in the UK with idiopathic normal pressure hydrocephalus. And in the US the figure is a staggering 1,600,000.

(See the paper by Tanaka, Yamaguchi, Ishikawa, Ishii and Meguro in Japan and the article by Rosell CM, Andersson J, Kockum K, Lilija-Lund O, Soderstrom L and Laurell K in Sweden. The papers are listed among the references at the end of this book.)

Only a very tiny percentage of these individuals have been accurately diagnosed as suffering from idiopathic normal pressure hydrocephalus. The vast majority of these individuals who have been diagnosed at all will have been diagnosed as suffering from Alzheimer's disease or some other form of dementia or from Parkinson's disease. Many individuals, of course, will not have been given a diagnosis at all but will have been simply labelled 'old'.

A second way of measuring the incidence of normal pressure hydrocephalus is to look at the incidence of the disease among long-stay patients. The incidence of idiopathic normal pressure hydrocephalus is said to be around 14% among long-term patients in care homes, nursing homes and other residential centres – whether or not they have dementia. This figure suggests that in a small general nursing home with 20 patients, there are likely to be three patients who have idiopathic normal pressure hydrocephalus who could be treated and, possibly, cured. In a larger institution, specialising in the care of patients with Alzheimer's disease or some other form of dementia, the figure is likely to be much greater.

A third way of measuring the incidence of normal pressure hydrocephalus is to look at the number of people suffering from dementia in general and then look at studies where attempts have been made to assess the number of patients who have been misdiagnosed.

It is now generally agreed among experts that one in eight individuals over the age of 65 will have Alzheimer's disease (and, before they die, one in three individuals will develop some form of dementia). And it is also agreed that Alzheimer's patients make up between 50% to70% of all those suffering from dementia. This would suggest that between one in four and one in six individuals aged 65 or over are suffering from dementia.

The big question here is: 'How many of the patients diagnosed as suffering from irreversible, untreatable dementia are actually suffering from a disease (idiopathic normal pressure hydrocephalus) for which a cure is available?'

The Hydrocephalus Association in the United States estimates that there are 700,000 adults in America who have idiopathic normal pressure hydrocephalus but that only a fifth of these patients have been diagnosed. The remainder have been misdiagnosed as suffering from Alzheimer's, some other dementia or Parkinson's disease. Available scientific evidence suggests that the majority of the four fifths of the 700,000 who are undiagnosed could be treated and restored to good health.

So, according to the Hydrocephalus Association in America, there are 560,000 patients in the US who have idiopathic normal pressure hydrocephalus but who do not know it, have not been diagnosed or treated and who are being left to die, untreated and without hope. The figures for the UK and other countries are undoubtedly similar. If we extrapolate from the American figures, it would suggest that there are a quarter of this number in the UK (a total of 140,000) who have treatable idiopathic normal pressure hydrocephalus but who have been misdiagnosed as suffering from an untreatable dementia. Given the fact that idiopathic normal pressure hydrocephalus is very little known in the UK I suspect that the true figure is considerably higher than this.

There are currently an estimated 45 million people around the world who have been diagnosed as suffering from dementia or Alzheimer's Disease. There is little doubt that several million of them have been wrongly diagnosed and, if they had been correctly diagnosed, could have been cured. The key thing to remember is that normal pressure hydrocephalus can be cured with a single, relatively simple surgical procedure. And the bottom line is that patients with dementia, who are confined to a hospital or nursing home or to bed in their own homes, can become independent again if they are treated.

Very few specialist studies have been done to measure the incidence of idiopathic normal pressure hydrocephalus among patients in 'assisted living facilities' or 'extended care facilities' but the results which exist show that between 9% and 14% of the patients studied had idiopathic normal pressure hydrocephalus.

Chapter Four

Why are patients with idiopathic normal pressure hydrocephalus often mistakenly diagnosed as suffering from other disorders such as Alzheimer's disease, other dementias or Parkinson's disease?

'Many people go undiagnosed and untreated because the symptoms of normal pressure hydrocephalus can mimic Alzheimer's disease, Parkinson's disease and other neurological or spinal disorders that can occur in adults as they age,' says Michael Williams, a neurologist and director of the Adult Hydrocephalus Center at the Sandra and Malcolm Berman Brain and Spine Institute at Sinai Hospital of Baltimore in Maryland, US.

The size of this scandal is difficult to comprehend and as the number of people in their 60s and beyond increases, so the number of people with treatable idiopathic normal pressure hydrocephalus will increase proportionally.

Idiopathic normal pressure hydrocephalus was first identified in 1965. No one has any idea how many people have been misdiagnosed since then. Because of ignorance among doctors and nurses, idiopathic normal pressure hydrocephalus is rarely diagnosed and so it is invariably categorised as a 'rare disease'. (These days, nurses demand and expect to be given clinical authority and to be treated as principals in the diagnostic process; consequently they must share the responsibility when things go wrong.)

But idiopathic normal pressure hydrocephalus is not a rare disease. On the contrary, when doctors and nurses are aware of the disorder, it is remarkably common. Moreover, it is the only form of dementia which is curable.

Chapter Five

Six case histories

1. Professor Emeritus of Hepatology Harold O Conn MD FACP of the Yale University School of Medicine in the US developed problems with walking shortly after retiring. He was 68-years-old when the symptoms started. They gradually became more pronounced. Dr Conn was diagnosed by colleagues in the department of neurology at Yale University as suffering from 'Parkinson's disease like syndrome'. Dr Conn's wife noticed that her husband was losing his sense of humour and his ability to concentrate. He also developed double incontinence. Three more eminent neurologists were consulted and they diagnosed a variant of Parkinson's Disease. They offered a poor prognosis. At a follow up appointment, five years after they made their diagnosis, they predicted that the cerebral atrophy would continue and that the professor's symptoms would get worse. They also said that the condition was untreatable. Nine years after the initial symptoms had appeared, when he was 77-years-old, Dr Conn could barely walk. He was then seen by a neurologist in another state. The new neurologist made a diagnosis of idiopathic normal pressure hydrocephalus. When 60 mls of cerebrospinal fluid was removed, Dr Conn made an immediate improvement. And after shunt surgery was performed, Dr Conn improved permanently. He had had the disease for 10 years and had repeatedly been wrongly diagnosed by specialists working in one of the world's premier medical schools.

2. A 40-year-old widow and housewife, Mrs LCB, was referred from the General Outpatient Department of the Jos University Teaching Hospital to the hospital's psychiatric unit in May 2014. She had eight weeks history of recurrent vomiting, recurrent headaches, fearfulness and withdrawal. She had been in good health up until the start of that period of illness. The patient's headache was described as generalised, throbbing and non-radiating and it was mildly

relieved with analgesics. There was some dizziness and blurring of vision. She had some fever, felt weak and could walk only with support. Since the patient had recently witnessed gunshots in Nigeria, an initial diagnosis of Post-Traumatic Stress Disorder was made. Two weeks after admission to the psychiatric unit, the patient had a convulsion and also complained of progressive weakness of her lower limbs and of urinary incontinence both during the day and at night. Her speech also became irrational and she had visual hallucinations. At that point, a diagnosis of Generalised Tonic Clonic seizure was made. A CT scan revealed idiopathic normal pressure hydrocephalus. The patient had a ventriculo-peritoneal shunt surgery. Following the surgery the patient did well and all symptoms subsided. The patient was able to walk with minimal support. The doctors looking after this patient reported that in their experience, idiopathic normal pressure hydrocephalus can be relieved successfully with a shunt implanted surgically to drain excess cerebrospinal fluid. The details of this patient were reported in the Journal of Neurological Disorders. The article was entitled Normal Pressure Hydrocephalus with Onset Following a Traumatic Experience. The author of the article was Aishatu Yusha'u Armiya'u of the Department of Psychiatry, Jos University Teaching Hospital, Jos, Plateau State, Nigeria.

3.

Bob Fowler was so convinced that he was dying that he wrote his own obituary. He had, in his own words, 'been to doctor after doctor after doctor with absolutely no positive results'. For nine years, Mr Fowler increasingly suffered with trouble walking, memory problems and difficulty controlling his urination. Eventually, Mr Fowler developed severe dementia, had to stop working and was confined to a wheelchair. After some years, his wife began making plans to put him in a nursing home. Finally, Mr Fowler met a doctor who recognised that he had idiopathic normal pressure hydrocephalus. After surgery, Mr Fowler literally got up out of his wheelchair and resumed his life. The change was dramatic. 'All of a sudden I felt fantastic,' he said. 'I'm 74-years-old now, and I'm doing things I wouldn't have dreamed of doing anytime during my 60s.' Mr Fowler went back to work, started playing golf, driving his car and spending time with his family. This case history was discovered on the internet.

4.

Retired dentist Milton Newman suffered for 15 years with loss of memory and concentration. Mr Newman's symptoms started when he was about 55-years-old. 'Reading a book was difficult because I couldn't remember what happened 10 pages back. And later on, conversation was difficult because I'd forget what people would say.' Eventually Mr Newman was diagnosed as suffering from Alzheimer's disease. He regarded the diagnosis as a death sentence. Finally, after years of suffering, Mr Newman met a doctor who diagnosed idiopathic normal pressure hydrocephalus. Surgery reduced the symptoms immediately. 'I felt like the old Milton,' said Mr Newman. This case history was discovered on the internet.

5.

A 70-year-old woman suffered a gradual onset of gait disturbance and later on developed dementia and occasional urinary incontinence. For two years, her mental problems got worse and her ability to walk deteriorated to the point where she was unable to walk and care for herself at home. She became a hospital patient in Norway after she had first noticed her symptoms. A CT scan showed ventricular enlargement out of proportion to the cerebral atrophy. When a lumbar puncture was performed, it was found that the CSF pressure was raised. When a shunt operation was performed, the patient gradually improved and a year later she was able to live normally at home. Her dementia had improved considerably, her urinary incontinence had disappeared and her gait was almost normal. This case history was discovered on the internet.

6.

The final year of my mother's life was a living nightmare.

And yet if the incompetent staff at two hospitals in Devon had been a little more alert, and a little less arrogant, my mother could have been cured. She had idiopathic normal pressure hydrocephalus but, despite her obvious symptoms, and much prompting, the diagnosis was ignored. Her treatment can only be described as uncaring and barbaric.

I still find my mother's story enormously difficult to relate but it should provide all of us, patients, relatives, doctors, nurses and administrators, with valuable lessons and so I have included it here.

My mother's story begins when, in October 2004, she had difficulty in walking. When she was admitted to Royal Devon and Exeter hospital in Exeter, she was thought to need extensive physiotherapy to help her walk again. She was mentally alert. Suddenly, in November 2004, after a rapid deterioration, it was decided that my mother was suffering from terminal cancer with metastases. She was not considered healthy enough for palliative radiotherapy and was described, by her consultant oncologist, as 'frail, confused, bedbound and dependent'. She had to be catheterised because she was incontinent. The idea of rehabilitation was abandoned because of her alleged terminal cancer. A neurologist who assessed her mental state reported that my mother did not know where she was and had failed to recognise the doctor. She was given the usual simple mental test (date of birth and so on) and scored 0 out of 10. My father was telephoned at home and told that my mother was terminally ill with cancer and that there were metastatic deposits in her spine, lungs and possibly liver. It was thought that her mental condition could be caused by secondaries in her brain.

No one knew what sort of cancer she was suffering from or where the primary was situated but the oncologist who had made this diagnosis told me that my mother either had cancer of the breast or the lungs with secondary deposits and that she was too weak for treatment. 'That's the nature of the beast', said the consultant.

My wife (who has no formal medical training) made the diagnosis by keying my mother's symptoms and signs into a search engine. Antoinette came up with several different diagnoses. From the short list she produced, we both agreed that idiopathic normal pressure hydrocephalus was by far the most likely diagnosis. The disease fitted my mother's symptoms perfectly. She had an unusual wide legged walk. She had a tendency to fall. And she had urinary incontinence. She was also showing signs of dementia. These are precisely the symptoms shown by patients with idiopathic normal pressure hydrocephalus.

We repeatedly suggested the diagnosis of idiopathic normal pressure hydrocephalus but doctor after doctor rejected it until it was too late. They seemed bizarrely desperate to settle on every possible diagnosis that wasn't the right one, and in retrospect I can only suspect it was because they knew little or nothing about idiopathic normal pressure hydrocephalus.

Moreover, is it possible that my mother's condition was ignored or treated superficially because of her age? She was 83 when her symptoms started but had been in excellent health up until that point. A couple of weeks before the onset of her illness, my mother and father had visited my wife and me in Paris. While in France, my mother had been alert and perfectly mobile. She had walked 15 miles one day when we had strolled down from Sacre Coeur in Montmartre to the area around the Eiffel Tower, taking an enjoyable roundabout route.

After her illness began, I repeatedly contacted my mother's family doctors in Budleigh Salterton in Devon and I spoke and wrote regularly to the vast variety of doctors at the hospital in Exeter. On a number of occasions I suggested that my mother was suffering from idiopathic normal pressure hydrocephalus but the doctors and nurses seemed concerned only to produce diagnoses which were untreatable and terminal. Only at the end, when it was too late to do anything, did they agree that she had all along been suffering from idiopathic normal pressure hydrocephalus.

Sadly, I do not think that this attitude is uncommon. Medical staff take little interest in patients who are over 60 years of age, and this lack of concern has been endorsed and encouraged by politicians. The United Nations has introduced Sustainable Development Goals which allow governments and health services to discriminate against anyone over the age of 70 on the grounds that people who die when they are over 70-years-old cannot be said to have died prematurely and so will not count when a nation's healthcare is being assessed. The Sustainable Development Goals give politicians the authority to ignore the health needs of citizens who have reached their 'three score years and ten' and who are regarded by society's accountants as an economic burden. Indeed, there is, regrettably a widespread assumption in hospitals everywhere that anyone who is over the age of 70 (and, in some cases, 60) must simply learn to live with their problems and adapt to changes which are simply an inevitable part of the ageing process. The Liverpool Care Pathway, which entitles doctors and nurses to withhold food, water and essential treatment from patients who are over the age of 65 and who are, therefore, regarded as an expensive nuisance is still used as a guideline by many doctors and nurses and hospital bureaucrats who are searching for ways to clear 'blocked beds' and reduce nursing costs.

On Sunday 21st November 2004, we noticed that my mother's urine bag was red. There was clearly blood in her urine. A nurse had changed the catheter bag several times without bothering to report to anyone that the urine in the bag was red with blood. Or perhaps they hadn't noticed. I reported the blood, and a doctor put my mother on amoxicillin for a urinary infection. After the blood appeared in the urine, the cancer specialist told me that my mother had secondaries in her kidneys. By the 30th November, the urine was clear and the bag was no longer red. The diagnosis of cancer secondaries in the kidneys was never withdrawn, though it too was completely wrong.

My mother stayed in the Exeter hospital for the next few months.

(The Royal Devon and Exeter hospital where my mother was treated so appallingly is a teaching hospital where medical students are turned into doctors.)

Numerous consultants saw my mother and decided that there was nothing to be done. Just about every different doctor came up with their own favourite diagnosis but although my wife and I repeatedly suggested that my mother might be suffering from idiopathic normal pressure hydrocephalus, no one seemed keen to accept this solution. No one really seemed to know anything much about it. My mother's symptoms now seemed to defy diagnosis. She managed to get out of bed occasionally but was unsteady on her feet. And she had developed a rather strange way of walking with her feet wide apart.

Idiopathic normal pressure hydrocephalus is not something of which GPs are aware. But it is the sort of thing teaching hospital doctors really should know about. I had never seen a patient with it. The hospital doctors looking after my mother listened politely to my suggestion that they consider idiopathic normal pressure hydrocephalus but immediately dismissed the idea and stuck with their neoplastic madness. There was never a shred of evidence in support of that diagnosis.

The care my mother received was appalling. She spent virtually all her time in bed, becoming steadily weaker. We couldn't move my mother to a private hospital because she had not yet been diagnosed, and clearly a private hospital would not have the investigative wherewithal. When I asked if I could send in private physiotherapists, I was told that I could not. The nurses on the ward did not seem to have heard of the danger of deep vein thrombosis or the need to avoid pressure sores by moving patients around.

On occasion, my mother would throw off all her clothes and we would have to rush to draw the screens while we fought to pull the bed covers over her. The nurses didn't come because the ward had been designed in such a way that from the nurses' station it was difficult if not impossible for nurses to see what was happening on the ward.

Once, I sat beside my mother's bed when two nurses arrived and one said: 'Have you had a drink this morning? 'Yes thank you,' said my mother, who had been officially declared demented and mentally incompetent. 'Right.' said the nurse. She wrote this information down on the fluids chart she was carrying. The cold cup of tea was standing, untouched, on the bed table in front of my mother. If we hadn't helped her drink, I firmly believe that my mother would have died of dehydration. Maybe that was the idea.

At one point during her stay in the Exeter hospital, at my urging, my mother had a diagnostic lumbar puncture and a quantity of cerebrospinal fluid was removed. Immediately afterwards she improved noticeably. For a day or two she seemed stronger and her mental function began to improve. It seemed to me that the improvement was significant and suggested that there had been too much fluid around my mother's brain. It seemed likely that the lumbar puncture, by removing some of the fluid, had reduced the pressure and alleviated her symptoms. Maybe the diagnosis of idiopathic normal pressure hydrocephalus was correct after all.

The doctors at the hospital all dismissed my suggestion and insisted that the improvement was simply a coincidence. What would a former GP and a writer of books know about these things? No one actually patted me on the head but it felt as though they had done so.

It was not until just before she died that my mother was finally diagnosed as suffering from idiopathic normal pressure hydrocephalus. Here is what one large medical textbook says: 'To help with the diagnosis, doctors do a spinal tap (lumbar puncture) to remove excess cerebrospinal fluid. If this procedure relieves symptoms, idiopathic normal pressure hydrocephalus is likely, and treatment is likely to be effective.' There are very few devastating diseases that can be cured so cheaply, so quickly and so permanently.

On Monday 25th April 2005, the neurology registrar at the Royal Devon and Exeter hospital announced that my mother's prognosis was bleak. The hospital staff still hadn't made a diagnosis. The cancer diagnosis had been forgotten. I was told that six neurologists and numerous other consultants had seen her and that every conceivable test had been done. The registrar told me that it would be difficult to find a nursing home capable of looking after her for in addition to her physical paralysis, she was again diagnosed as suffering from dementia. I was told that this could be vascular or a consequence of possible encephalitis. It seemed clear that my mother needed to stay in hospital for the rest of her life.

On Tuesday 26th April 2005, my mother was, at my request, moved to Budleigh hospital so that my father, who lived in Budleigh Salterton, could visit more easily. For six months he had visited the Exeter hospital once or twice a day to feed my mother (who would otherwise have almost certainly starved to death). I also wanted my mother out of the hospital in Exeter because I wasn't terribly impressed by the nursing care she had received. If I had to choose two words to describe the hospital care, they would be 'apathetic' and 'neglectful'. The hospital in Budleigh was clearly what used to be a cottage hospital – suitable for providing nursing care for local patients.

On Wednesday 27th April 2005, at 9.00 p.m., someone from Budleigh hospital telephoned my father (who was 85 at the time) and asked him when he would be moving his wife out of the hospital. My mother had been in the Budleigh hospital for just slightly more than 24 hours. No one there had made any attempt to make a diagnosis.

My father was startled and shocked by the suddenness and timing of the telephone call asking him when he would be moving my mother out of the hospital. He got the impression that the hospital was planning to send my mother home for him to look after by himself. She was incapable of doing anything for herself. She was now doubly incontinent, required nursing on a ripple bed and had been diagnosed as demented. She had to be kept in a bed with cot sides so that she didn't fall onto the floor. On the odd occasion when she tried to feed herself, she ended up with food everywhere – with the result that both she and the bed had to be changed. My mother was so incapable of moving by herself that the nurses had a hoist and a bed lift fitted to the bed so that they could move my mother around and in and out of bed. It took two nurses to move her up the bed. She needed constant nursing attention.

My wife and I were in France when my mother was moved to the hospital in Budleigh. We came straight back and visited the hospital on Thursday the 28th April.

Within five minutes of my arriving at my mother's bedside, a nurse asked me to go to the sister's office where a rude and aggressive nurse demanded to know when my mother would be leaving the hospital. My mother had, by then, been in the hospital for no more than 48 hours. I found the questioning cruel, unfeeling and inhumane.

My father, who had been in a state of shock, now became depressed as a result of the hospital's attitude. Up until Monday the 25th April, my father had hoped that he would eventually be able to have my mother back home or that, at the very least, he would be able to take her out of the hospital for trips in a wheelchair. He had been making plans to buy a motorised chair and a suitable vehicle so that he could do this. He had retained the hope that someone would find a way to treat my mother and produce some improvement in her symptoms.

When I spoke to the nurse at Budleigh Hospital on 28th April 2005, I was told that an assessment had been done and that my mother was considered fit to move out of the hospital. I was also told that she was now regarded as mentally alert. My mother had, according to Budleigh Hospital, been cured from her dementia within two days. She had received no new treatment. The nurse admitted that my mother needed nursing care but insisted that mentally there was nothing wrong with her. The hospital had, she told me, already applied for an enforcement order to have my mother removed from the hospital. I was shocked by their ruthlessness.

In reality, there had been no change whatsoever in my mother's condition. Several neurologists at Royal Devon and Exeter hospital had already agreed that my mother was suffering from severe dementia and though it turned out that they had missed the primary diagnosis, there wasn't much doubt that a diagnosis of dementia was accurate.

I complained about the fact that my father had been rung at home the evening before but the nurse didn't seem to think that there was anything wrong with that. She didn't apologise. I wanted to know just how ill you had to be to be in hospital these days. I felt overwhelmed with guilt. I had arranged for my mother to be moved to the Budleigh Hospital so that my father could visit more easily. And now they wanted to throw her out. But where could we take her? I went back to sit by my mother's bed. As I sat down, my mother looked up and pointed to a stranger on the other side of the ward. 'Is that Vernon over there?' she enquired. We were living a nightmare. She didn't know who I was. She didn't recognise my wife. And she often wasn't sure who my father was. When I talked to her, my mother didn't even know that she was in hospital. Somewhere in the hospital a bell rang. 'There's someone at the door,' she said.

A day or two later someone at the Budleigh hospital threatened to send my mother home in an ambulance, even though they knew that my father could hardly look after himself let alone care for someone who needed intensive nursing care. My mother was, said one NHS employee, terminally but not finally terminally ill. It was the first time I'd heard the phrase.

My father was devastated. 'What do I do if they send her home?' he asked. 'Don't answer the door,' I told him. 'Don't let them into the house. Call me.'

I was telling my father to refuse to let the ambulance men bring my mother into the house.

It was awful, just bloody awful. If the plan was to put us under pressure it was working very well. I'd never seen my father so distraught.

My mother's GP at the time agreed that we would not be able to find a local nursing home capable of looking after her. No one at the Budleigh hospital seemed to me to give a damn about what happened to my mother as long as she wasn't their responsibility.

As far as I am aware, no one made the slightest attempt to make a diagnosis during the time my mother was in the Budleigh Hospital. Since they didn't want to nurse her and they didn't do any diagnostic tests, it's difficult to see the point of the hospital – apart from providing employment for the staff.

On the 11th May, I had to attend a meeting at Budleigh hospital to discuss my mother's expulsion from the hospital. I was told that the hospital did not have enough beds and desperately needed to get rid of my mother. There were four people at the meeting: two members of the nursing staff, someone who looked like an administrator and my mother's GP. The meeting was held in a completely empty ward. There were plenty of beds, all empty, and it seemed to me that this wasn't the first time the empty ward had been used for a meeting. If the hospital was short of anything it was patients, not beds.

The meeting lasted an hour and it turned out to be one of the most unpleasant hours of my life. It was not a meeting where the words 'compassion' and 'caring' figured large. I have been grilled by some of the country's toughest television and radio interviewers. I have given evidence in the House of Lords and the House of Commons but nothing prepared me for this. For a solid hour, the four of them battered at me to take my mother out of the hospital. They used every manipulative and emotional trick in the book. I quickly realised that no one there cared a damn about my mother or my father. They just wanted to get rid of a patient who seemed likely to be a long-term expense. This was business. I was still desperate to try to find a diagnosis. I was still trying to support my father. I was grieving for my mother who no longer even recognised me.

I was told that my mother would be better off in a nursing home and that the hospital didn't have any long-stay beds. I was told that they needed her bed for other patients (no one seemed to see the irony in the fact that the meeting was being held in a completely empty ward) and that my father would be better off if my mother was elsewhere. They didn't explain how this could be when there was no nursing home for miles that would be able to cope with her needs.

At the end of the meeting I was told that they couldn't agree to my mother staying in the hospital and that she had to leave. I left the meeting and went back to my mother's bedside. She was still unable to move. She still didn't know who she was or where she was. She didn't know who I was. She was still faecally incontinent. She still had a catheter in her bladder to collect her urine. She still had to be fed. She still couldn't walk or even wash herself. But according to the hospital staff she was fine and mentally alert.

Ageism is the new racism: no respect, no consideration, no courtesy, no dignity, no caring.

For several weeks after that, my father didn't dare visit my mother at all. He was frightened that he would again be pressured by the staff to move my mother. He didn't know where he could take her. Overwhelmed with grief he was now also tortured by guilt and anxiety.

Another mental assessment was done on my mother. It was a sick joke. The assessor asked my mother what I did for a living. My mother thought for a while. 'He's a teacher,' she said at last. She didn't know who I was, let alone what I did for a living. 'That's close enough,' answered the assessor putting a tick in another box. My mother was declared mentally competent.

Later that day my father was sitting by my mother's side when the vicar called. My mother told him they were waiting for a train. The vicar thought it was a joke but my mother was serious. She kept asking my father why the train wasn't there and why there were dogs fighting in the vicinity. My mother now didn't recognise my father (to whom she had been married for over 60 years) or know what he'd done for a living. She didn't even know who she was or where she was. She held her head a good deal though and it was clear that she was having constant headaches. (No one at the hospital realised that these were caused by the increase in the amount of fluid surrounding her brain.)

On the 27th July, I attended another meeting in Budleigh Hospital. This time there were nine people there representing the hospital and the NHS. My mother's GP was there, together with two nurses, a 'continuity care manager', an 'acting leading continuity nurse', a 'hospital care manager', a 'discharge facilitator', a representative of the administrators and a representative from Exmouth social services.

Someone began by saying that they all had my mother's best interests at heart. Someone else said they were delighted to report that my mother was much better and was improving. I asked them why, if this was the case, they weren't giving her any occupational therapy or physiotherapy. No one had an answer to this. I asked them how they had managed to produce this miracle without any treatment. I wanted to know how a woman who had been officially declared terminally ill and demented, and in need of constant care, had suddenly become 'physically capable and mentally alert' after a few weeks in a small town hospital. No one had any answers.

In fact, of course, when the final diagnosis was made it was quite clear that my mother could not possibly have shown any physical or mental improvement. She was suffering from idiopathic normal pressure hydrocephalus which was steadily getting worse. NHS staff who said that my mother had recovered and was no longer demented and could be discharged were lying because they wanted to throw her out of the hospital.

When I pointed out that my mother needed intensive nursing care, a continuity care manager claimed, to my utter astonishment, that catheters, hoists and ripple beds were not medical equipment. I asked him what would count as medical equipment. He said a ventilator would count as medical equipment. The phrase 'final stage terminal illness' was now used. And again I heard the phrase 'terminally, terminally ill'. I asked how they knew that a patient was terminally, terminally ill and was told that they could tell this through liver and kidney deterioration. I asked if they had done any tests to check on this, and it was generally agreed that they couldn't remember whether any such tests had been done.

I have no idea why nine people wasted a good chunk of a day on such a pointless meeting. I hate to think what it must have cost. It occurred to me as I sat there that if they were all sacked there would be plenty of money left for looking after patients. I told them that the bullying had won and that we would take my mother out of the hospital so that they could have yet another empty bed.

The truth was that my father couldn't bear it any longer. The staff at the Budleigh Hospital were making us feel so unwelcome, and harassing us so much, that we had no choice but to move my mother. As far as the NHS was concerned, it was all about money. They wanted to avoid the cost of looking after my mother – even though they had a moral and legal responsibility to do so.

We found a private nursing home in Exmouth where for a vast weekly fee a week my mother had a private room which seemed crowded with three adults visiting. If a hotel had offered us the room we would have walked out in disgust. Naturally, there were now no attempts to make a diagnosis.

My father sold his home and bought a small house near to the nursing home so that he could visit regularly.

27

Towards the end of her life, we were visiting my mother in the nursing home when Antoinette pointed out that my mother had a swollen, bulging eye. (My wife had, by this time, more knowledge of idiopathic normal pressure hydrocephalus than the entire NHS medical staff in Devon.)

The diagnosis was now beyond doubt. My mother had a bulging eye because of the pressure inside her skull.

In idiopathic normal pressure hydrocephalus, the pressure within the skull remains normal because the expanding fluid volume compresses and destroys brain tissue. When the brain cannot be compressed any more then the fluid pressure must rise.

I contacted my mother's new GP and asked him to arrange for my mother to go back into Exeter hospital. I don't believe that he or any of the nursing home staff had noticed anything wrong.

In the Royal Devon and Exeter Hospital, the doctors at last confirmed the diagnosis of idiopathic normal pressure hydrocephalus. It was the diagnosis we'd offered them months earlier. Numerous consultants (including several neurologists), countless junior hospital doctors, two GPs and several dozen nurses all missed the diagnosis. If they'd acted within days or even weeks of her being admitted to hospital then they could have saved her life. We watched my mother die a terrible, slow death. She died because the doctors failed to make the diagnosis until it was too late.

Note: I did think about cutting this section (which is, I know, rather lengthy) but I know about my mother's experiences at first hand and I think it is important that readers understand just how uncaring health professionals can be when dealing with elderly, demented patients. I have named the hospitals concerned so that readers can be sure that the facts described here are perfectly accurate.

Chapter Six

How can idiopathic normal pressure hydrocephalus be diagnosed?

The principle symptoms of idiopathic normal pressure hydrocephalus are: a wide legged, unsteady gait, a tendency to fall a good deal (commonly falling backwards), incontinence (usually urinary but double incontinence sometimes occurs) and dementia. Other symptoms and signs may include headaches. Patients usually appear slow thinking and have impaired memory. They may lose their inhibitions and behave inappropriately in company – saying or doing things that are completely out of character. Patients have difficulty in starting and carrying out tasks, find it hard to focus and lose motivation. They tend to sleep a good deal.

Because other types of dementia may produce similar symptoms, or symptoms which can be confused with these, or because the dementia may be such a dominant symptom that it overwhelms the others, it is dangerous to try to make a diagnosis of idiopathic normal pressure hydrocephalus from the symptoms alone.

As a starting point, most doctors investigating dementia and suspecting idiopathic normal pressure hydrocephalus will perform a scan; either an MRI scan or a CT scan. MRI is safe and painless and takes at least half an hour. MRI uses radio signals and a powerful magnet to create a picture of the brain. It will show if the ventricles are enlarged and will provide information about the surrounding brain tissue. An MRI scan will also evaluate the flow of cerebrospinal fluid. An MRI scan provides more information that is likely to be used in making a diagnosis of idiopathic normal pressure hydrocephalus. A CT scan creates a picture of the brain using X-rays and a special scanner. It is safe, reliable, painless and quicker than an MRI and it will show if the ventricles are enlarged or if there is any obvious blockage.

A scan of the brain may show that there is excess cerebrospinal fluid and that the ventricles within the brain are enlarged. Unfortunately, these findings are not pathognomonic – though they certainly suggest that a diagnosis of idiopathic normal pressure hydrocephalus is possible if not probable.

The most accurate way to make a diagnosis is to do a lumbar puncture (also known as a spinal tap) and to remove some of the excess cerebrospinal fluid from around the spinal cord and the brain. If there is an improvement within three or four days after a lumbar puncture has been done and some fluid removed then the diagnosis of idiopathic normal pressure hydrocephalus is likely. And there is a real chance that the patient's symptoms can be improved.

It is usually wise to allow some cerebrospinal fluid to drain for a few days while evaluating the patient.

If there is a clinical improvement after 30 mls or so of fluid have been removed then there will probably be a good response if a shunt is put into place.

However, the fact that there is no improvement after some cerebrospinal fluid has been removed does not mean that a diagnosis of idiopathic normal pressure hydrocephalus is impossible. It may still be worth putting in a shunt – especially if other signs and symptoms suggest that it might help. It is worth remembering that idiopathic normal pressure hydrocephalus is one of the few diseases masquerading as dementia (and by far the most common) which can be treated effectively. Some patients improve (occasionally dramatically) if CSF fluid is removed. But other patients show no improvement after fluid is removed. Whether or not a patient shows improvement after fluid removal does not have any impact on whether or not a shunting operation will produce a good result.

As you might expect from the name of the disease, the cerebrospinal fluid pressure is usually normal in patients with idiopathic normal pressure hydrocephalus. (Since there is more fluid, you'd expect the pressure to be higher. But it isn't, probably because the fluid gradually enlarges the space it takes up by making the ventricles larger.)

When a shunt has been placed in situ, it will probably be necessary to adjust the rate at which fluid is draining out. If too much fluid has been allowed out then the patient may develop a headache. The outflow of cerebrospinal fluid can be adjusted without extra surgery. If a shunt is not draining away enough fluid then the first symptoms to recur will probably be related to walking. The recurrence of a walking problem may mean that the shunt is not working properly or that it needs to be adjusted so that more fluid drains out. It is important to remember that far too little research has been done into idiopathic normal pressure hydrocephalus and, in a sense, every patient is an experiment.

There are other tests which may be done to find out whether a patient has idiopathic normal pressure hydrocephalus.

One of these is the infusion test in which the outflow of cerebrospinal fluid is measured. This test assesses the degree to which the absorption of CSF back into the bloodstream has been blocked.

Another test is to measure the intracranial pressure. A small pressure monitor is inserted through the skull into the brain or the ventricles to measure the intracranial pressure. Unfortunately, this is not necessarily diagnostic since, of course, patients with idiopathic normal pressure hydrocephalus will not usually have raised intracranial pressure.

Finally, there is a test known as isotopic cisternography which involves injecting a radioactive isotope into the lumbar subarachnoid space through a spinal tap. This test allows the absorption of CSF to be evaluated over several days. This test is not particularly often used because it is complicated, and does not reliably predict whether a patient will respond well to shunt surgery.

If a patient is to be properly diagnosed and treated then, in addition to the GP or primary care physician, advice will be needed from a neurologist and a neurosurgeon. There will be two important decisions to make: is the patient suffering from idiopathic normal pressure hydrocephalus and are they likely to benefit from a shunting operation.

Chapter Seven

How can idiopathic normal pressure hydrocephalus be treated?

The aim of treatment is to get rid of the excess cerebrospinal fluid which has accumulated and which is doing the damage. In order to remove the excess fluid, a small piece of plastic tubing (known as a shunt) is placed in the ventricles of the brain and run under the skin to the abdomen where the fluid drains away and is gradually absorbed into the body. This mechanically simple procedure is known as ventriculoperitoneal shunting.

Alternatively, the tubing can lead from the brain to the right atrium of the heart. This is known as ventriculoatrial shunting.

Whatever type of shunt is used, the opening pressure of the valve can be adjusted in order to avoid side effects created by removing too much or too little fluid. This is usually done with the aid of a small magnet which controls the valve's setting and which can be rotated with the aid of a stronger magnet.

Recently, surgeons have begun to perform lumboperitoneal shunt surgery which, it seems, may prove to be safer. (One end of the shunt tube is placed in the spine and the other end in the abdominal cavity) A study reported in 2015 suggested that the lumboperitoneal approach is effective. According to Professor S Chabardes, Head of the Functional Stereotactic Unit at the Department of Neurosurgery of the Joseph Fourier University, Grenoble, France: 'This shunt might be better accepted and tolerated by the patients.'

Whatever type of operation is performed there seems no doubt that this sort of treatment definitely works.

Professor G L Lenzi, from the Department of Neurology of La Sapienza, Rome, has stated that: 'patients who had surgery significantly improved motor and non-motor symptoms compared to the non-surgical patients'.

Whatever type of shunt is used, a good response is usually obtained within a few hours of the procedure being performed, with the patient being able to walk more easily and being less incontinent. There is also often a significant improvement in mental function.

The earlier the diagnosis is made, and the earlier treatment is initiated, the greater the chances that the patient's mental capacities will improve. Some early studies suggested that only patients in the early stages of the disease benefitted but more recent studies have shown that putting in a shunt will result in a noticeable or marked improvement in between 70% and 86% of patients who have quite severe symptoms. On the whole, experts have concluded that more than 80% of those having surgery experience improvement. The age of the patient does not seem to have any effect on the outcome. There can be risks with this type of surgery but if the diagnosis has been made then patients and relatives may well feel that the risks are worth taking. Risks in medicine must always be related to the seriousness of the illness involved. If a patient is going to die then even a risky procedure is worth trying.

Much of the important research into idiopathic normal pressure hydrocephalus has taken place in Sweden and scientists there have developed a way of measuring cerebrospinal fluid dynamics. Artificial cerebrospinal fluid is added and the resultant resistance is measured. The greater the resistance the more likely it is that the patient will benefit from treatment. The scientists also measure the effects of removing 50 mls of cerebrospinal fluid. If tests show an improvement in the patient's ability to think and to move after the removal of the fluid then good results from surgery are much more likely.

Sometimes, patients who have had a good deal of cerebrospinal fluid removed (because a shunt is overdraining, for example) may develop headaches. When this happens, the headache can be minimised by using an adjustable shunt.

Chapter Eight

What is the prognosis when idiopathic normal pressure hydrocephalus is diagnosed and treated?

Once the shunting operation is performed, patients with idiopathic normal pressure hydrocephalus will often make quite remarkable recoveries.

It is well known that the human brain can recover after a stroke (in which the tissue may be starved of oxygen by a blood clot or starved of oxygen and compressed by a bleed) and that it is possible for stroke victims to recover lost mental and physical skills for many months after an incident. Similarly, there is no reason why the brain cannot make a remarkable recovery after the traumas of idiopathic normal pressure hydrocephalus although, of course, progress is likely to be faster and more complete when the diagnosis is made at an early stage and the treatment started early.

Around 80% of patients benefit from the shunt surgery offered as treatment and it is worth remembering that this figure will probably be higher in patients who have good general health and lower in patients who have poor general health and who are suffering from other problems such as diabetes or high blood pressure. The patient who is exceptionally frail and weak is unlikely to do as well as the patient whose only health problem is the idiopathic normal pressure hydrocephalus for which he is being treated.

According to a paper entitled 'Long-term outcome in 109 adult patients operated on for hydrocephalus', which was written by Tisell M, Hellstrom P, Ahl-Borjesson G, Barrows G, Blomsterwall M, Tullberg M, Wikkelso C. and published in the British Journal of Neurosurgery in 2006, 79% of patients who responded to a questionnaire after a medium follow-up time of 4.2 years reported that they still felt improved and 60% had 'persisting observable improvement of gait, living conditions, bladder function and need of sleep'.

It is clear that the majority of patients with idiopathic normal pressure hydrocephalus who are diagnosed and treated with surgery have a beneficial outcome.

It is worth remembering that patients who have the condition and are not treated will continue to deteriorate and will eventually die.

There are, sadly, some (including many in political positions of authority) who do not believe in providing health care for those who have passed a certain age. However, from a purely financial point of view this is nonsense.

Unless society is preparing to introduce mass euthanasia for all patients suffering from dementia then curing patients, and enabling them to live practical, profitable and useful lives must be preferable in every conceivable way (including financial) to leaving them to be dependent upon 24 hour nursing care, whether that care is provided professionally or by relatives.

Chapter Nine

Why do doctors so rarely diagnose idiopathic normal pressure hydrocephalus?

Idiopathic normal pressure hydrocephalus was identified in 1965 but even today, over a century later, there is still very little about the disease in the medical journals, and medical textbooks devote very little space to the problem. I have in front of me a large medical book which contains over 2,000 pages of closely printed text. Less than half of one page is devoted to idiopathic normal pressure hydrocephalus. I have seen several major medical textbooks which make no mention at all of the disease.

One major textbook, containing nearly 4,000 pages, also devotes just half of one page to normal pressure hydrocephalus and, after dismissing the disease in such a remarkably cavalier fashion, adds that 'this disorder accounts for up to 6% of dementias'. Since there are reckoned to be at least 50 million dementia sufferers in the world, that would mean that there are approximately 3 million patients in the world with idiopathic normal pressure hydrocephalus – most of them untreated. And this is a disease which can be cured.

If you have never heard of a disease, or you know very little about it, then you are unlikely to think of it when you see a patient suffering from what appears to be a form of dementia. Sadly, the easy thing for a doctor to do is to make a diagnosis of Alzheimer's disease and abandon the patient to a life of inevitable, remorseless decline. If normal pressure hydrocephalus is untreated then the path of the disease will match that of Alzheimer's disease and no one, least of all the doctor, will question the doctor's diagnosis.

Doctors who have heard of normal pressure hydrocephalus say that it is a rare disease. The fact is, however, that it isn't so much a rare disease as a rarely diagnosed disease. If doctors aren't aware of it and don't look for it then they will never see it.

An important and revealing study done in Sweden showed that the majority of doctors considered themselves to have 'poor knowledge' about the symptoms of normal pressure hydrocephalus.

I would suspect that in the UK and the US the word 'very' could reasonably be placed before the words 'poor knowledge'. My own experience suggests that a majority of doctors have never heard of the disease and therefore never think of it when making a diagnosis of dementia or Alzheimer's disease.

The failure to diagnose normal pressure hydrocephalus has undoubtedly resulted in millions of patients living out the final years of their lives requiring full-time nursing care. How many countless million years of productive life have been wasted? And how many relatives and friends have suffered unnecessarily as they have watched their loved ones die slowly and with a steadily increasing loss of cerebral function?

The pure financial cost of this failure by the medical profession is impossible to estimate accurately. It is estimated that the cost of dementias to the UK is £26.3 billion a year. The country could, without doubt, save many billions of pounds a year by diagnosing and treating patients with idiopathic normal pressure hydrocephalus.

Finally, it is important to remember that relatively little research has been done into this disease and although we do know that it is far commoner than is generally appreciated, there is a desperate need for more research into the causes of the disease as well as into ways of making a rapid diagnosis and new ways to treat the disorder quickly and efficiently.

Chapter Ten

Why has idiopathic normal pressure hydrocephalus not been investigated more thoroughly?

It is not possible to estimate the emotional and social cost of Alzheimer's disease and dementia. The heartbreak of watching someone you love lose their mind is difficult to explain.

If just 1% of the patients currently languishing in hospitals, nursing homes and private homes could be cured then much heartache would be avoided.

It is no exaggeration to say that many millions of patients who require 24 hour nursing care could be returned to useful, independent, productive and rewarding lives if those patients with idiopathic normal pressure hydrocephalus were correctly diagnosed and not merely dismissed as suffering from an incurable dementia. It cannot be said too often that this is a common condition and it can be cured.

Vast amounts of money are spent by medical researchers – sometimes on disorders which affect very few patients. Vast amounts of publicity is given to disorders which are genuinely rare.

So, why is idiopathic normal pressure hydrocephalus so little known?

And why is so little effort put into researching the disorder?

Part of the answer is that very little money is spent on researching or publicising disorders which affect the elderly. Disorders which affect those over 60 are regarded as unglamorous and therefore not worth the attention of politicians, doctors, nurses or journalists.

But the main answer, I'm afraid, lies in the way that medical research is conducted.

Most medical research is organised and paid for by drug companies looking for new products to sell. Doctors and scientists hoping to be given grants will usually look for a drug solution to any problem because they know that the best way to obtain drug company money is to offer a possibly valuable and profitable therapeutic solution to a chronic problem. Similarly, many charities have links with drug companies. And they too will be keen to make it clear that money given to them will be spent on searching for a solution which can be patented and then prescribed or sold over the counter.

There is no need to find a pharmaceutical solution to idiopathic normal pressure hydrocephalus because we already know how to cure the disease. A relatively simple one-off operation will provide a long-term cure. There is no opportunity for a researcher or a charity to offer a drug company a profitable outcome if they help pay for a research programme into the disease.

And so little or no research is done.

And since many of the world's medical journals are effectively controlled by drug companies (which provide the advertising which keeps the journals alive) there are few articles drawing attention to a disease which the medical profession has more or less forgotten.

So idiopathic normal pressure hydrocephalus remains almost unknown.

Chapter Eleven

What relatives and friends can do if they suspect someone might have idiopathic normal pressure hydrocephalus

Whenever a diagnosis of Alzheimer's disease or any other type of dementia is made then it is wise to seek a second or third opinion. Similarly, when a diagnosis of Parkinson's disease is made another opinion should be sought. Idiopathic normal pressure hydrocephalus is often missed but it can be treated with spectacular, life-saving results.

'People shouldn't assume that all dementia is incurable Alzheimer's and that their situation is hopeless,' says neurosurgeon Ann Marie Flannery, a member of the joint guidelines committee of the American Association of Neurological Surgeons and Congress of Neurological Surgeons.

Michael Williams, the neurologist, says that 'the literature in the past 15 years shows that if you conduct the right tests and select the right patients, the likelihood of benefit is quite high and the risk of harm is quite low.'

Writing as the relative of a patient who had the disease, and having seen the effects of idiopathic normal pressure hydrocephalus far closer than I would have liked, I would say that the risks of performing the shunting operation are always worth taking if a diagnosis of idiopathic normal pressure hydrocephalus is probable or even possible. When a patient is demented, bed bound and doubly incontinent the potential upside is dramatic and the guaranteed downside is of limited consequence.

And the simple fact is that everyone will benefit if more patients are properly diagnosed. Treating idiopathic normal pressure hydrocephalus in the elderly population will reduce health care expenditure dramatically, and make hospital beds available for more acute patients. The cost of caring for patients with dementia is now said to cost more than cost of caring for all patients with cancer and heart disease. Diagnosing, treating and curing the hundreds of thousands who have idiopathic normal pressure hydrocephalus would save (literally) billions a year.

It is in all our interests to put more time, energy and money into investigating idiopathic normal pressure hydrocephalus and doing more to educate the public, the medical profession and the nursing profession about a disease which is a surprisingly common cause of dementia and the only common cause of dementia which can be treated and cured.

Selected References

Conn HO. Normal pressure hydrocephalus: a case report by a physician who is the patient. Clin Med 2007 June; 7 (3) 296-9

Blomsterwall E, Svantesson U, Carlosson U, Tullberg M, Wikkelso C. Postural disturbance in patients with normal pressure hydrocephalus. Acta Neurol Scand 2000 Nov; 102(5) 284-291

Hellstrom P, Edsbagge M, Archer T, Tisell M, Tullberg M, Wikkelso C. The neuropsychology of patients with clinically diagnosed idiopathic normal pressure hydrocephalus. Neurosurgery 2007 Dec; 61(16): 1219-26; discussion 27-28

Marmarou A, Bergsneider M, Relkin N, Klinge P, Black PM. Development of guidelines for idiopathic normal pressure hydrocephalus: introduction. Neurosurgery 2005 Sep: 57(3 Suppl): 51-3, discussion ii-v

Takeuchi T, Kashara E, Iwasaki M, Mima T, Mori K. Indications for shunting in patients with idiopathic normal pressure hydrocephalus presenting with dementia and brain atrophy (atypical idiopathic normal pressure hydrocephalus). Neurol Med Chir (Tokyo) 2000 Jan; 40(1):38-46; discussion -7

Eklund A, Smielewski P, Cahmbers I, Alperin N, Malm J, Czosnyka M, et al. Assessment of cerebrospinal fluid outflow resistance. Med Biol Eng Comput 2007 Aug; 45(8):719-35

Wikkelso C, Andersson H, Blomstrand C, Lindqvist G, Svendsen P. Normal pressure hydrocephalus. Predictive value of the cerebrospinal fluid tap-test. Acta Neurol Scand. 1986 Jun; 73(6): 566-73

National Institute of Neurological Disorders and Stroke. NINDS Normal pressure hydrocephalus informationpage. 2011

Adams R.D, Fisher C.M, Hakim S, Ojeemann RG, Sweet WH. Symptomatic occult hydrocephalus with normal cerebrospinal fluid pressure. New England Journal of Medicine 273(3) 117-126

Krauss JK, Faist M, Schubert M, Borremans JJ, Lucking CH, Berger W. Evaluation of gait in normal pressure hydrocephalus before and after shunting. Gait Disorders 2001 (pp301-309) Philadelphia PA: Lippincott Williams and Wilkins

Ropper, AH, Samuels MA. Adams and Victor's Principles of Neurology 2008, McGraw Hill

Younger DS. Adult normal pressure hydrocephalus. Motor disorders 2005 (pp581-584) Lippincott Williams and Wilkins

Tamaris, A, Toma AK, Kitchen ND, Watkins LD, Ongoing search for diagnostic biomarkers in idiopathic normal pressure hydrocephalus. Biomarkers in Medicine 2009 Dec: 787-805

Marmarou A, Bergsneider M, Klinge P, Relkin N, Black PM. The value of supplemental prognostic tests for the preoperative assessment of idiopathic normal pressure hydrocephalus Neurosurgery 2005 Sept 57 (3 Suppl): S17-28, discussion ii-v

Marmarou A, Young HF, Aygot KA. Estimated incidence of normal pressure hydrocephalus and shunt outcome in patients residing in assisted living and extended care facilities. Neurosurgical Focus 2007 Apr 22(4) 1-8

Vanneste J, Augustijn P, Dirven C, Tan WF, Goedhart ZD. Shunting normal pressure hydrocephalus: do the benefits outweigh the risks? A multicentre study and literature review. Neurology 1992 Jan 42(1) 54-9

Poca MA, Mataro M, Matarin MdM, Arikan F, Junque C, Sahuquillo J. Is the placement of shunts in patients with idiopathic normal pressure hydrocephalus worth the risk? Results of a study based on continuous monitoring of intracranial pressure. Journal of Neurosurgery 2004 May, 100(5) 855-866

Brean A, Eide PK. Prevalence of probable idiopathic normal pressure hydrocephalus in a Norwegian population. Acta Neurologica Scandinavica 2008 July. 118(1) 48-53

Tanaka N, Yamaguchi S, Ishikawa H, Ishii H, Meguro K. Prevalence of possible idiopathic normal pressure hydrocephalus in Japan: the Osaki-Tajiri Project. Neuroepidemiology 2009 32(3) 171-175

Malm J, Graff-Radford NR, Ishikawa M, Kristensen B, Leinonen V, Mori E, Owler BK, Tullberg M, Williams MA, Relkin NR. Influence of comorbidities in idiopathic normal pressure hydrocephalus – research and clinical care. A report of the ISHCSF task force on comorbidities in INPH. Fluids and Barriers of the CNS. Biomed Central 2013. 10.22

Johansson E, Ambarki K, Birgander R, Bahrami N, Eklund A, Malm J. Cerebral microbleeds in idiopathic normal pressure hydrocephalus. Fluids and Barriers of the CNS. Biomed Central 2016. 13:4

Armiya'u AY. Normal pressure hydrocephalus with onset following a traumatic experience. J.Neurol Disord (2014) 2:184

Kazui H, Miyajima M, Mori E, Ishikawa M. Lumboperitoneal shunt surgery for idiopathic normal pressure hydrocephalus (Sinphoni-2): an open label randomized trial. Lancet Neurology 2015; 14:585-594

Svein IB, Tore AM, Torbjorn H. Reversible dementia in idiopathic normal pressure hydrocephalus: a case report. Scandinavian Journal of Primary Health Care 1999; 17:1 22-24

Hakim S, Adams RD. The special clinical problem of symptomatic hydrocephalus with normal cerebrospinal fluid pressure: observations on cerebrospinal fluid hydrodynamics. J Neurol Sc 1965; 2:307-27

Galassi R, Morreale A, Montagna P, Sacquegna T, DiSarro R, Lugaresi E. Binswanger's disease and normal pressure hydrocephalus. Clinical and neuropsychological comparison. Arch Neurol 1991; 48:1156-9

Fisher CM. Hydrocephalus as a cause of disturbances of gait in the elderly. Neurology 1982:32 1358-63

Bergeson SE, Gjerris F, Serensen SC. The resistance to cerebrospinal fluid absorption in humans. A method of evaluation by lumbo-ventricular perfusion, with particular reference to normal pressure hydrocephalus. Acta Neurol Scand 1978; 57: 88-96

Anderson M. Normal pressure hydrocephalus BMJ 1986; 293: 837-8

Vanneste JAL, Augustijn P, Dirven C, Tan WF, Goedhart ZD. Shunting normal pressure hydrocephalus: do the benefits outweigh the risks? A multicentre study and literature review. Neurology 1992; 42:54-9

Hughes CP, Siegel BA, Coxe WS, Gado MH, Grubb RL, Coleman RE et al. Adult idiopathic communicating hydrocephalus with and without shunting. J Neurol Neurosurg Psychiatry 1978;41: 961-71

Friedland RP. Normal pressure hydrocephalus and the saga of the treatable dementias. JAMA 1989; 262: 2577-81

Cox J, Knox J, Brocklehurst G. Normal pressure hydrocephalus. J Am Geriatr Soc 1988:36:650

Folstein MR, Folstein S, McHugh PR. Mini-mental state: a practical method for grading the cognitive state of patients for the clinical. J Psycho Res 1975; 12:128-98

Benson DF. Neuroimaging and dementia. Neurol Clin 1986; 4:341-53

Vanneste JAL. Three decades of normal pressure hydrocephalus: are we wiser now? J Neurol Neurosurg Psychiatry 1994; 57: 1021-5

Clarfield AM. The reversible dementias: do they reverse? Ann Intern Med 1988; 109:476-86

Wyper D, Pickard JD, Matheson M. Accuracy of ventricular volume estimation. J Neurol Neurosug Psychiatry 1979; 42: 345-50

Coleman V. Do doctors kill more people than cancer? European Medical Journal 2011

Kizu O, Yamada K, Nishimura T. Proton chemical shift imaging in normal pressure hydrocephalus. Am J Neuroradio 2001 Oct; 22:1659-1664

Rosell CM, Andersson J, Kockum K, Lilija-Lund O, Soderstrom L, Laurell K. Fluid Barriers CNS. Abstracts from Hydrocephalus 2015; 12 (Suppl1):O55.

Tisell M, Hellstrom P, Ahl-Borjesson G, Barrows G, Blomsterwall M, Tullberg M, Wikkelso C. Long-term outcome in 109 adult patients operated on for hydrocephalus. British Journal of Neurosurgery 2006; 20(4):214-21

Printed in Great Britain
by Amazon

48483581R00033